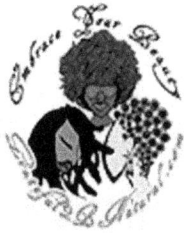

Grateful 2 B Natural

The Naturalista's Do It Yourself (DIY) Recipe Book

Recipes for Beautiful Hair, Gorgeous Skin

and Healthy Body

Nyla Al-Mujaahid

The Naturalista's Recipe Book– Recipes for Fierce Natural Hair, Glowing Skin & Beautiful Body

By Nyla Al-Mujaahid

Grateful 2 B Natural, Inc

Published in the United States by Grateful 2 B Natural, Inc

Copyright © 2013 by Nyla Al-Mujaahid

Al-Mujaahid, Nyla

The Naturalista's Recipe Book– Recipes for Fierce Natural Hair, Glowing Skin & Beautiful Body / Nyla Al-Mujaahid

ISBN: 978-0989082402

Also by Nyla Al-Mujaahid

Unloc'ed- The Journey From Locs to Free-Flowing Natural Hair without Chopping Them Off

Seminars by Nyla Al-Mujaahid

Natural Beauty Academy
Natural Beauty Business Academy
Dynamik D.I.V.A. Academy

Meet Nyla online and receive free training at
NylaAlMujaahid.com

Dedicated to my husband & best friend, my wonderful children, my naturalicious mother & sisters as well as the Fierce Naturalistas & Dynamik D.I.V.A.s. You Rock!

Contents

Styling Products

Cleansers

Moisturizers

Snacks

Beverages

Preface

Going through the "Natural Journey" can be a road of learning, growing and most definitely one of change. One thing that's certain is that there will be questions.

"What products do I use on my natural hair?
"What foods are best for my skin, hair and body?
"What are 'cones', sulfates, etc? Are they truly bad for me?
"Do I have to give up the things I love to have the body, skin & hair that I want?

Of course the list goes on. There are many questions that we face when it comes to taking care of ourselves, so going natural, (whether it be natural hair or natural foods) the same rings true.

One way to make the process simple is to Do It Yourself or DIY. I know that it can seem overwhelming with our already busy lives to make our own products or go 'back in the day' and make our foods from 'scratch'. That is why this book will give you easy to follow recipes for hair care, skin care as well as recipes that will please your palate and enhance your beauty from the inside out.

I wanted to provide a guide to help take the guess work out of what products to use when we are 'going natural'. I also wanted to provide a source that will help us take charge of what is going into and on our bodies and be more preventive when it comes to health and beauty. A true beauty is a healthy beauty. One who takes care and pride in her health and appearance. *True beauty is not fake or phony. When we put the right things in and on our bodies we lessen*

the chance of having to go to extremes to 'look beautiful'. Our skin glows so we don't have to put on

heavy make-up or 'push broom' eyelashes. Our hair grows so we don't have to wear lace front wigs or excessive extensions.

For naturalistas of color, there are not many books or guides out there that are "for us, by us" that give us insight on how to care for our "natural" selves. I'm talking about from what we eat, to how we look as well as how to nurture positive relationships. This recipe book is the first of many installments of the Grateful 2 B Natural Naturalistas series of books.

So enjoy the recipes that follow and take charge when it comes to taking care of you.

Embrace your beauty. Be Grateful 2 B Natural!

Nyla

Please note: Before you start any type of diet, plan or program please consult with your physician. I trust that we are all smart individuals, so do not in any way take what you read in this book as medical advice. The recipes and tips in this book are for informational purposes and the reader is responsible for his or her own actions

How to Get the Most From This Book

Ok naturalistas, of course this is a recipe book so it would be simple to say, "Follow the recipes and enjoy". Although I believe in simplicity, I won't tell you that.

Use this book as a guide. Make the recipes, but put your own spin on them as well. You know what you like and what may benefit and/or harm you. (I have food as well as medicinal allergies, so I rarely ever follow anything 'by the book'.)

Make sure you read the "Important Nutrients' section and make a point to marry them into your diet as well as any products you make for your skin and hair.

Most importantly, enjoy your creations. You are taking charge of taking care of you. No artificial preservatives, additives, flavoring or color. Au' Naturale.

Oh, one more thing. Get together with friends and family and share your creations. Trust me, I've tried a number of these recipes on my family and friends and they were pleasantly surprised with the food and felt lavishly pampered with the products. Sharing is caring. Encourage positive change for better health and beauty! ☺

Introduction

When it comes to having beautiful hair, glowing skin as well as a healthy gorgeous body, we must be mindful of what we put on as well as in them. It's not easy to read every label on every product we come across. It's time consuming and confusing, especially when we are trying to figure out the words that we are unable to pronounce.

What's even more brain-teasing is the question, "Where do the ingredients come from?" It seems as though we have to be scientists or chemists in order to make out what we are trusting in and on our bodies, hair and the like.

Do It Yourself or DIY, receives its fame from the phrase, "If you want it done right..." So, why do so many of us trust our health, whether it is hair health or body health, to those who only have dollars on the brain?

This recipe book started as an idea to help my fellow naturalistas really take charge of embracing their natural beauty. That is why there are three recipe sections in this book. Having healthy hair, healthy skin and a healthy body goes hand in hand. You cannot fully have one without the others.

The benefits of taking the DIY approach to your hair and body health are limitless. You know the ingredients of your products; you become savvier with your funds, you become more creative, less of a product junkie, and more in control of your life. I know it may sound like I'm reaching, but trust me, this and more happens when you take control of what goes in and on your body...and hair for that matter.

So, this recipe book is not just designed to give you a few recipes and tips to use on your skin, hair and whatnot. It's designed to help you embrace your natural beauty and take charge by being creative and responsible for what is important...yourself. Enjoy the recipes and if you haven't already, get serious about fully embracing your natural beauty.

Hair Care Recipes

These easy to prepare DIY natural hair care recipes are fitting for any naturalista, whether transitioning, brand new or a long-time Naturalista D.I.V.A. This section is broken down into three categories: Cleansing, Conditioning & Styling. The products you create will be able to save you time from label reading and looking through various products to find what's right for your hair as well as money spent on products that just don't cut it. I heard from a fellow curlfriend, "If I can't put it in my body, why should I put it in my hair?" It makes sense since our scalp absorbs the product we put in our hair.

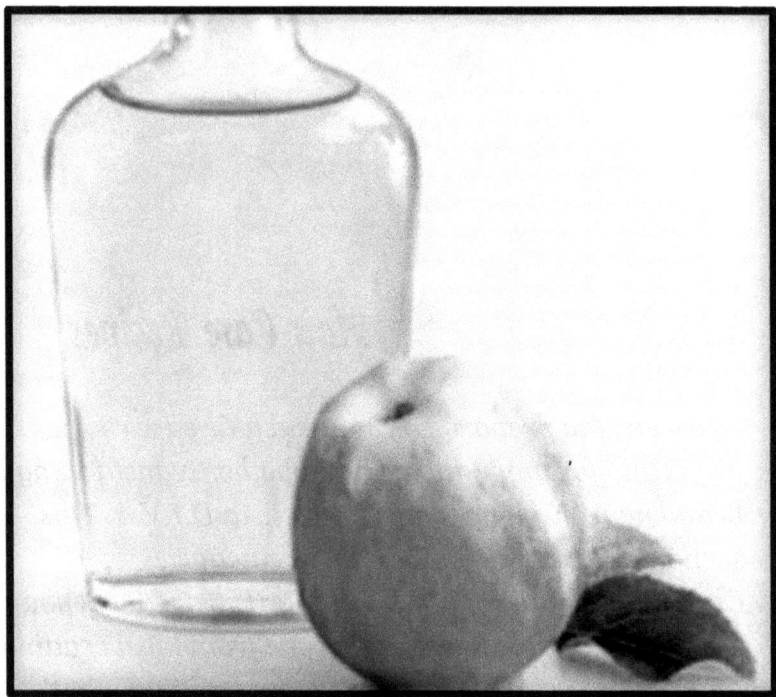

The health benefits of Apple Cider Vinegar or ACV are endless. Apple Cider Vinegar is known for removing product build-up on the hair & scalp

Cleansing Products

Chamomile Shampoo

Ingredients

6 organic chamomile tea bags

4 tablespoons pure soap flakes

1 1/2 tablespoons pure vegetable glycerin

Directions

Steep the teabags in 1 1/2 cups of boiled water for 20 minutes. Remove the tea bags and discard. Add the soap flakes to the tea and let stand until the soap softens. Stir in glycerin until well blended. Keep in a dark, cool place in a sealed bottle.

Natural Shampoo for Normal Hair

Ingredients

1/4 cup water

1/4 cup liquid castile soap

1/2 teaspoon organic sunflower oil or other light organic vegetable oil

Directions

Mix together all the ingredients. Store in a bottle. Use as you would any shampoo, rinse well.

Aloe Vera Shampoo for Dry Hair

Ingredients

1/4 cup liquid castile soap

1/4 cup organic aloe vera gel

1 teaspoon pure vegetable glycerin

1/4 teaspoon organic avocado oil or other light organic vegetable oil

Directions

Mix together all the ingredients. Store in a bottle and always shake well before using. Apply to hair and allow it to sit for a few minutes. Rinse well with cool water.

Baking Soda Clarifier for Heavy Product Build-Up

Ingredients

3 tablespoons baking soda

1 1/2 teaspoons creamy honey

1/4 teaspoon water

Cider Vinegar Clarifying Hair Rinse [see below]

Directions

Mix ingredients together to form a paste. Add additional water, a few drops at a time, if the mixture is too thick. Shampoo hair as usual. Apply mixture to hair and leave on for up to five minutes. Rinse hair as usual. Pour Cider Vinegar Clarifying Rinse through hair, do not rinse again [the cider vinegar scent will very quickly dissipate]. If your hair is "squeaky clean" apply a light leave-in conditioner. This is best used for first-time clarifying, by those who use a full line of hair products that include silicone that have left behind a heavy build-up, or those who clarify rarely.

Clarifying Cider Vinegar Hair Rinse

Ingredients

1/2 cup cider vinegar

1 1/2 cups cool water [the cooler the better]

Directions

Mix ingredients in an unbreakable bottle. Shampoo and rinse hair as usual. Pour vinegar rinse through hair, do not rinse again [the cider vinegar scent will very quickly dissipate]. You can apply a leave-in conditioner to ends if necessary. Ratio of vinegar to water may be adjusted according to the amount of clarifying needed or frequency of use. This rinse is probably the most popular homemade hair product; it will effectively remove product build-up from hair [including silicone] and leave it very soft and shiny.

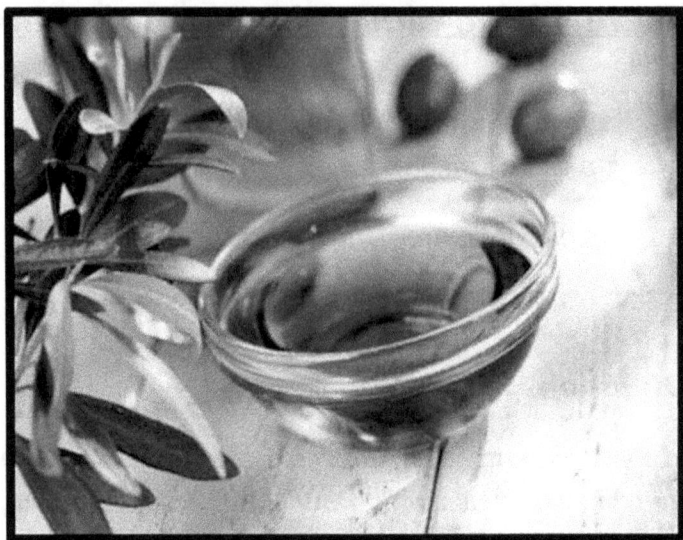

Olive oil makes a great hot oil treatment. Hot oil treatments are fabulous for restoring moisture to dry hair & scalp. They are also wonderful for 'pre-pooing' (a before shampoo treatment)

Conditioning & Moisturizing Products

Tropical Hair Conditioner

Ingredients

1 avocado

½ ripe banana

Organic coconut milk

Directions

Peel and pit avocado. Mash avocado with banana and slowly blend in coconut milk until smooth and the consistency of hair conditioner. Work through hair to ends. Rinse after 15 minutes and shampoo.

Avocado Deep Hair Conditioner

Ingredients

1 small jar of mayonnaise

1/2 avocado

Directions

Peel avocado and remove pit. Mix ingredients in a medium-sized bowl with a large spoon until it's a pudding like consistency. Smooth into hair being careful to work it to the ends. Use shower cap or plastic wrap to seal body heat in. Leave on hair for 20 minutes. For deeper conditioning wrap a hot, damp towel around your head over the plastic.

Nettle Hair Lotion

Ingredients

1 cup nettle leaf (not root)

Water

Directions

Simmer nettles in three cups of water. Strain. Rub into hair and scalp every other night for soft, shiny hair. Keep refrigerated.

Rosemary Hot Oil Hair Treatment

Ingredients

1/2 cup of organic dried rosemary

1/2 cup organic soybean oil or organic sunflower oil

Directions

Combine ingredients and heat until warm. Strain through a fine strainer or cheesecloth. Coat the entire head and hair with the oil mixture, working it through to the ends. Wrap hair in plastic wrap and wrap in a warm towel. Leave oil on hair for 15 minutes. Wash hair until oil is completely removed.

Hot Oil Treatment for Damaged Hair

Ingredients

1/2 cup organic soybean oil or organic sunflower oil

8 drops oil of sandalwood

8 drops oil of lavender

8 drops oil of geranium

Directions

Mix all ingredients well. Warm oil to a comfortable temperature and apply the mixture to damp hair. Wrap hair in plastic wrap and apply a hot towel for 20 minutes. Shampoo.

Lavender Rosemary Hot Oil Hair Treatment

Ingredients

1/2 cup organic soybean oil or organic sunflower oil

5 drops oil of rosemary

10 drops oil of lavender

Directions

Mix all ingredients well. Warm slightly and apply the mixture to damp hair. Wrap hair in plastic wrap and apply a hot towel for 20 minutes. Shampoo

Ginger Dandruff Treatment

Ingredients

Ginger root

1 teaspoon organic sesame oil

1 teaspoon lemon juice

Directions

Squeeze ginger root through press to obtain one tablespoon of juice. Mix all ingredients. Apply to scalp and let dry before shampooing. Repeat three times a week.

Quick Pre-Shampoo Hair Oil Treatment for Dry Ends

Ingredients

Olive oil

-Or-

Jojoba oil

Directions

Pour a small amount of oil into the palm of your hand. Rub palms together and gently apply to ends of hair. Shampoo as usual.

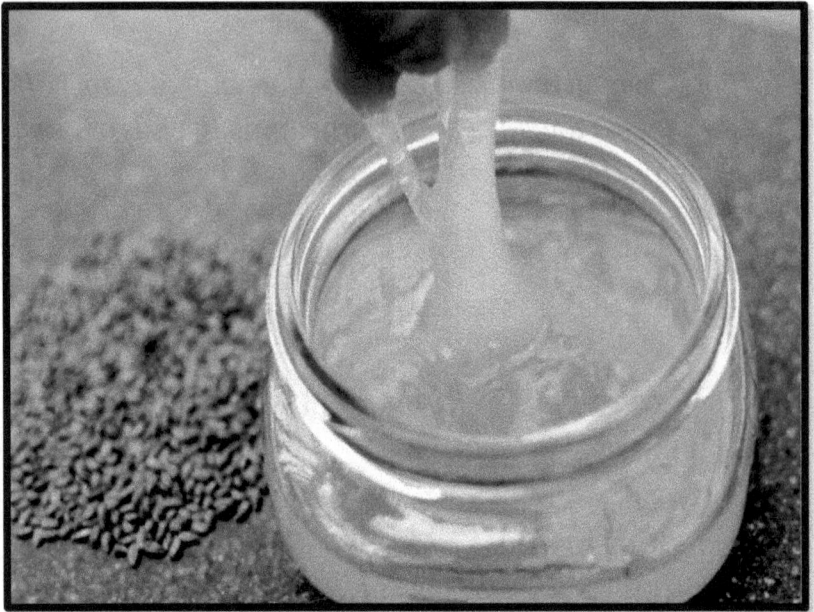

Flaxseed has many healthy benefits. It is high in Omega 3 fatty acids that are great for skin, hair & body and makes a great hair gel that keeps hair soft while giving a great hold.

Styling Products

Frizzy Hair Controller

Ingredients

1/2 cup good organic hair conditioner

1/4 cup pure honey

1 tablespoon organic almond oil

Directions

Mix all ingredients, blending well. Spray hair with water mister to dampen it. Work mixture through hair thoroughly. Leave on for 20 minutes. Shampoo.

Frizz Control for Curly Hair

Ingredients

1 small aloe vera leaf

Directions

Snip off end of leaf and apply a dollop of aloe vera gel to palm. Work through hair to ends.

Flaxseed Hair Gel

Ingredients

2 Tbsp Whole Flax Seeds
1 cup water
Pure Aloe Vera Gel, if desired
Few drops of essential oil for scent

Directions

Soak the flaxseeds overnight. This increases gel yield, increases ease of straining, and reduces cooking time. (This step is optional.) Combine the flaxseeds and water in a pan over high heat, stirring occasionally. Stir gently and constantly, when the mixture starts to boil. Reduce the heat to medium when the mixture's consistency turns into a thin, foamy jelly. When the seeds remain suspended in the jelly instead of sinking to the bottom of the pan, turn off the heat and drain the mixture through the strainer into the bowl. Add a preservative after the mixture has cooled slightly (optional). Add any desired ingredients, such as essential oils or aloe vera gel. Whisk the mixture to combine ingredients and break up any clumps. The gel should be about the consistency of egg whites. Pour the mixture into the container. Your gel is ready to use. Store in the refrigerator for maximum shelf life.

Natural Hairspray

Ingredients

1/2 orange

1/2 lemon

Directions

Chop fruit into small pieces and place in a pot with 2 cups water. (Peeling is unnecessary.) Boil until water is reduced by half. Cool, strain, and place in a spray bottle. Store in the refrigerator. Add more water to reduce stickiness, if desired.

Shea Butter Twist-Out Cream

Ingredients

1 Cup Shea butter

½ Cup Vegetable Shortening

2 Tbs Honey

Directions

Combine Shea butter, shortening and honey in a bowl. Mix well. Apply to damp or dry hair before twisting or braiding.

Skin Care Recipes

The recipes that follow are simple yet very effective for cleansing and moisturizing. The vitamins that are infused in these recipes are great for keeping bacteria at bay, increasing elasticity as well as shrinking pores.

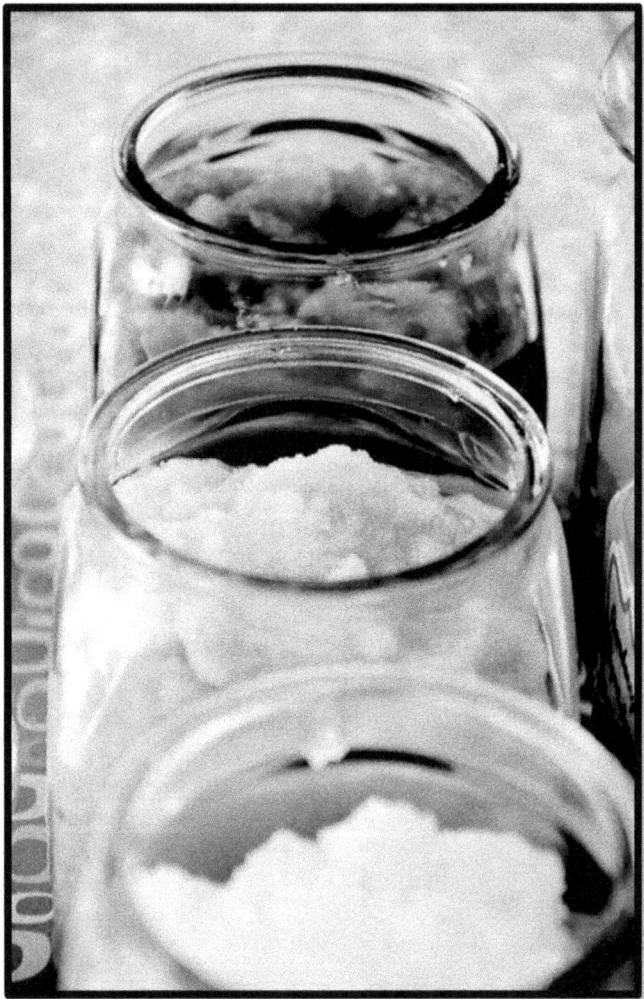

Coffee, sugar & salt scrubs are great skin cleansers

Cleansers

Milk & Honey Facial Cleanser

Ingredients

1 teaspoon dark organic Honey

1 tablespoon whole Milk (or cream)

Directions

Warm up the honey until it becomes runny (not too hot!) by putting it in a small glass or metal bowl which is immersed in hot water (or a few seconds in the microwave) Mix the honey and milk well

Skin Stimulating Facial Cleanser

Ingredients

1 ripe fresh Tomato

2 tablespoons Milk

1 tablespoon fresh Lemon juice

1 tablespoon fresh Orange juice

Directions

Put all the ingredients in a food processor and whizz it until it becomes a smooth watery substance. Keep refrigerated for a few days.

Chamomile Facial Cleanser for Sensitive Skin

Ingredients

4 tablespoons Cream

4 tablespoons Milk

2 tablespoons crushed dried Chamomile flowers

Directions

Put all ingredients in a double boiler and let them simmer for 30 minutes, but do not let it boil. Take it from the heat source and let it cool down for 3 hours, then strain it. Keep refrigerated.

Skin Brightening Facial Cleanser

Ingredients

1 slice peeled Apple

2 tablespoons Plain unflavored Yogurt, with active cultures

1 teaspoon Almond oil

1 teaspoon Lime juice

Directions

Put all the ingredients in a food processor and whizz them until you have a smooth watery substance. Store in refrigerator.

Facial Cleanser for Oily Skin

Ingredients

1/2 cup Buttermilk

2 tablespoons crushed Fennel seeds

Directions

Put the ingredients in a double boiler and let them simmer for 30 minutes. Take it from the heat source and let it steep and cool down for 3 hours, then strain it. Store in refrigerator

Deep Cleansing Honey Oatmeal Cleanser

Ingredients

3 tablespoons Oatmeal flour

1 tablespoon dark organic Honey

2 tablespoons Cream

2 drops Lavender oil

2 drops Juniper berry oil

Directions

Slowly warm up the cream in a double boiler (or 15-20 seconds in microwave) but do NOT let it boil. Add the honey and let it melt slowly. Then blend in the oatmeal *and leave it for 5 minutes. Now add the oils and blend it well*

Apply it to a warm, damp face and neck. Gently massage it on in circular movements. Rinse it off with warm water and end with a splash of cold; pat your skin dry

Exfoliating Cornmeal Scrub

Ingredients

2 tablespoons Cornmeal

1 tablespoon fresh Tomato juice

2 tablespoons Glycerin

1/2 glass Mineral Water

Directions

Mix all ingredients together until you have a smooth mixture. Warm this mixture up in a double boiler to thicken; do NOT boil it. Let it cool down before use; add extra mineral water if necessary

Gelatin Deep Pore Cleansing Mask

Ingredients

1 Tbs unflavored gelatin

1 Tbs milk

Directions

Mix gelatin and milk together in a glass or small bowl until gooey. Use small brush to apply to face. Let dry and peel or sloth off.

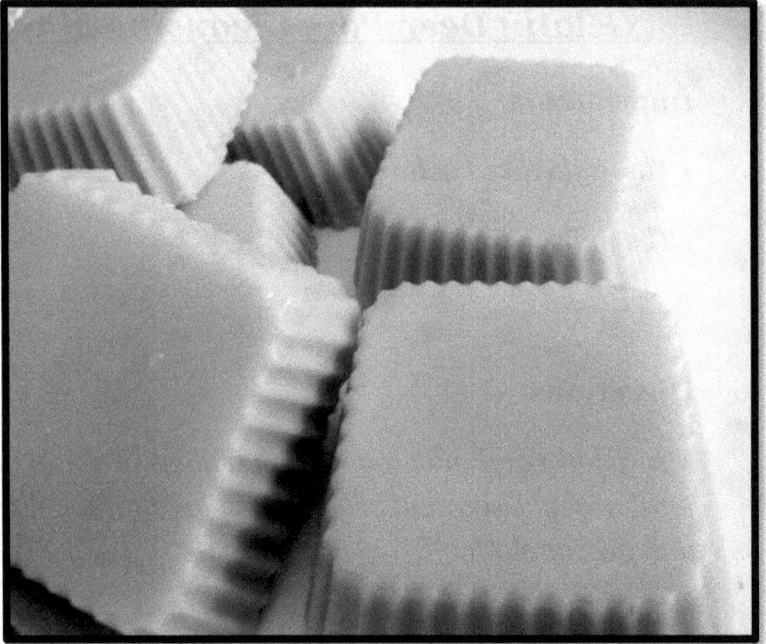

Lotion bars are a convenient way to moisturize on the go. They are easy to make and can last awhile. A no muss, no fuss way to keep your skin soft & supple

Moisturizers

Facial Moisturizer

Ingredients

Jojoba oil

Few drops essential oil of your choice

Small glass or plastic bottle

Directions

Mix the ingredients together. For every teaspoonful of jojoba oil, add 1 drop of essential oil. Pour into a bottle. Massage a few drops directly into your skin.

Moisturizing Lotion Bars

Ingredients

One part Beeswax

One part Almond Oil

One part Coconut Oil

Directions

In a large saucepan fitted with a double boiler, (or a bowl on top of a pot of boiling water) place the beeswax over medium heat. Once it is completely melted, add the almond oil to the double boiler.

Add the coconut oil. Allow it to melt completely. Remove the double boiler from the pan and put it on a towel; dry off any water that has accumulated on the bottom. Pour the mixture in to your mold of choice. Let bars set until cooled & solid.

Moisturizing Shea Butter Bars

Ingredients

One part Shea Butter

One part Grapeseed Oil

One part Coconut Oil

Directions

In a large saucepan fitted with a double boiler, (or a bowl on top of a pot of boiling water) place the shea butter over medium heat. Once it is completely melted, add the grapeseed oil to the double boiler. Add the coconut oil. Allow it to melt completely. Remove the double boiler from the pan (or bowl from pot) and put it on a towel; dry off any water that has accumulated on the bottom. Pour the mixture in to your mold of choice. Let bars set until cooled & solid.

Oatmeal Moisturizing Cream

Ingredients

1/4 cup of oatmeal/oats

3/4 cup of coconut oil

Few drops of rosemary oil

1 tbsp of olive oil

Directions

You will first need to finely ground the oatmeal to a powder/flour consistency. You can use a blender, food processor or a Magic Bullet type of appliance to finely ground the oats. Over low heat, melt the coconut oil until it

has a liquid consistency. Add a few drops of Rosemary
Essential Oil. Mix in the oatmeal flour until well
blended. Add olive oil and mix until well blended. Once
the ingredients are mixed, pour into a small storage
container. Let harden for several hours. Apply to
hands and skin as needed for skin softening,
moisturizing, soothing and healing.

Meal Time Recipes

The recipes in this section are delicious and supply vital nutrients for healthy skin, hair and body. These recipes are meatless because there is nothing wrong with a meat-free diet, however too much meat can cause problems which includes making our body more acidic when our body is healthier in an alkaline state.

You can, however add lean meat, chicken, turkey, fish, etc to the following recipes as you like. Experiment! Enjoy!

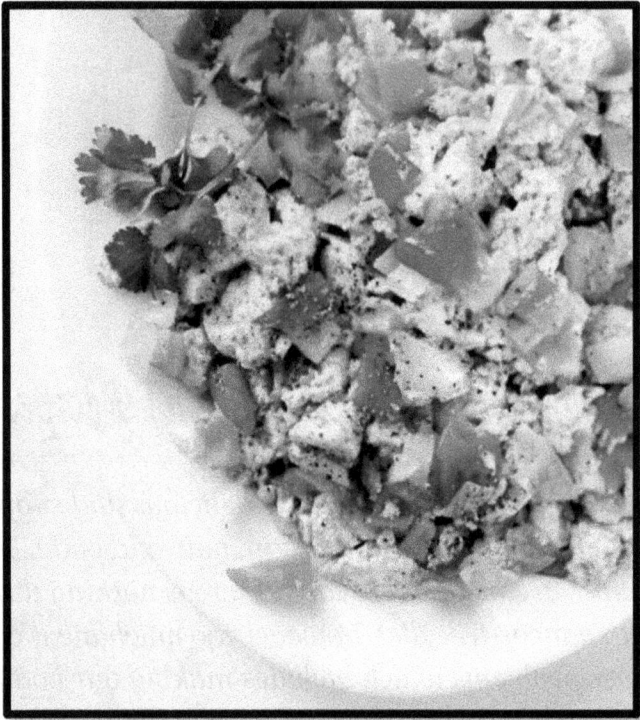

Tofu Scramble is a great way to start the day. It's packed with protein and you can add veggies & spices to design it to fit your taste

Breakfast Recipes

Multi-Grain Waffle Taco

Ingredients

1 Multi-grain waffle

1-2 Tbs Almond butter

1 Tbs Raisins, blueberries, sliced bananas, sliced strawberries or any fruit of your choice

1 Tbs Semi-sweet chocolate chips

Directions

Pop frozen waffle in toaster. Spread on almond butter. Add fruit and chocolate chips. Fold and go!

Raisin & Walnut Proatmeal

Ingredients

1 cup quick oats

¼ cup raisins

¼ cup walnuts

1 tsp cinnamon

¼ cup honey

2 tbs Vegetable protein powder

½ cup almond milk

Directions

Boil 2 cups of water in a pot. Add milk, oatmeal & honey. Cook oatmeal on medium heat for 5 minutes or until oats have expanded and oatmeal has reached a thick consistency. Add raisins, walnuts, cinnamon and protein powder. Stir well.

Avocado Breakfast Wrap

Ingredients

1 Avocado sliced

½ Tomato diced

1 Spinach wrap

¼ cup Black Beans (cooked or canned)

Scrambled firm tofu seasoned to your liking (or eggs, if you prefer)

Shredded Vegan cheese

Directions

Prepare tofu as you would scrambled eggs. To add the yellow color, add turmeric. Take your spinach wrap and pile on the goodies. Wrap it and enjoy!

*If you are using canned black beans and you prefer not to cook them, make sure you at least rinse them.

**Superfood Granola Parfait**

Ingredients

1 Scoop chia powder

8 oz Almond milk

1 Banana sliced and frozen

Blueberries

Granola

Directions

In a blender, blend almond milk and chia powder. Add sliced bananas and pulse until creamy. In a glass or mug, layer granola, berries and 'soft serve'.

*Chia is rich in vitamins, antioxidants and Omega 3 fatty acids. It's not just for Chia Pets ☺

Sweet Potato Proatmeal Casserole

Ingredients

1 cup quick oats

4 cups Almond milk

2 small or 1 medium sweet potato (peeled and chopped)

2 large ripe bananas

2 Tbs Chia powder

3 tsp Pure vanilla extract

4 Tsp honey

Nutmeg & Cinnamon to taste

Pecan Topping

2/3 cup chopped pecans

4 Tbs Vegan butter

4 Tbs unbleached all-purpose flour

½ cup brown sugar

Directions

Preheat oven to 350 degrees Fahrenheit. Boil sweet potatoes until fork tender. Drain and set aside. In a pot, add almond milk, oats and chia powder and whisk. Bring

to a boil for about 5-7 minutes. Mash cooked potato with banana and add to pot of oatmeal mixture. Cook on low heat for a few minutes.

Make topping by mixing pecans, butter, flour and brown sugar together well.

Butter baking dish and transfer oatmeal/potato mixture to dish. Add pecan topping and bake uncovered for 20 minutes. After 20 minutes set oven to Broil. Broil for a few minutes, watching carefully as not to burn topping. Remove from oven and serve.

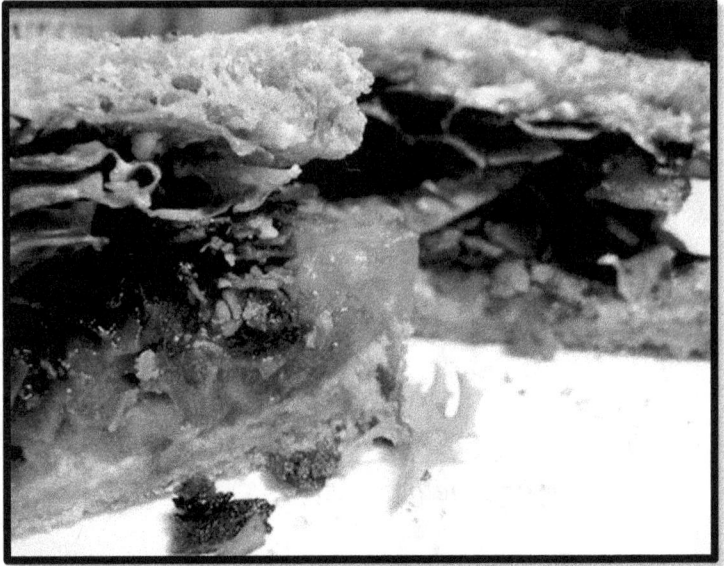

A vegan BLT made with coconut. Yes, the bacon or 'facon' as I call it is made from coconut. Even if you do not like coconut (I don't) you may enjoy this (I did ☺)

Lunch Recipes

Black Bean & Yellow Rice Bowl

Ingredients

1 Cup Cooked Black Beans

1 Cup Cooked Basmati Rice

2 Tsp Goya con Azafran

½ Avocado diced

½ Tomato diced

2 Tsp Grapeseed oil

Directions

Add Goya con Azafran, Grapeseed oil and Basmati rice to bowl. Stir until rice is coated and yellow. Toss in other ingredients.

Black Bean & Sautéed Veggie Pocket

Ingredients

¼ Cup Sliced Green Pepper

¼ Cup Sliced Red Pepper

¼ Cup Sliced Red Onion

¼ Cup Cooked Black Beans

2 Tbs Grapeseed or Olive Oil

¼ Cup of Fresh Spinach

1 Pita Pocket

Shredded cheese of your choice

Directions

Heat oil in skillet. Add peppers and onion and cook until tender, tossing frequently. Slice pita in half and add spinach, beans and veggies. Top with cheese.

Vegan BLT

Ingredients

3 ½ Cup Shredded coconut or flakes (unsweetened)

1 Tbs Liquid smoke

2 Tbs Tamari Soy Sauce

2 Tbs Honey

1 Tbs Sesame oil

Tomato

Kale

2 Slices of whole grain bread (toasting optional but recommended- yum!)

Directions

Preheat oven to 350 degrees Fahrenheit. Prepare the Vegan bacon buy combining coconut, Liquid Smoke, honey, Tamari and sesame oil in a bowl. Mix until coconut is coated well. Place 'bacon' on a cookie sheet and bake for 10 minutes. Stir and bake for another 5 minutes or until a nice dark brown.

Build your sandwich and enjoy!

Whole Grain Veggie Pizza

Ingredients

Whole Grain tortilla

1 Avocado mashed

½ Red Pepper sliced

½ Green Pepper sliced

½ cup Mozzarella Cheese (or more if you like)

1 cup Spinach

1 cup Black Beans

Directions

Spread mashed avocado on tortilla. Sprinkle on cheese. Add spinach, peppers and black beans. Enjoy!

Black Bean Lettuce Wraps

Ingredients

Boston lettuce leaves

Black beans (canned or cooked)

Cheddar Cheese

Diced Tomatoes

Diced Avocado

Directions

Wash lettuce leaves. Pile on ingredients. Wrap and enjoy!

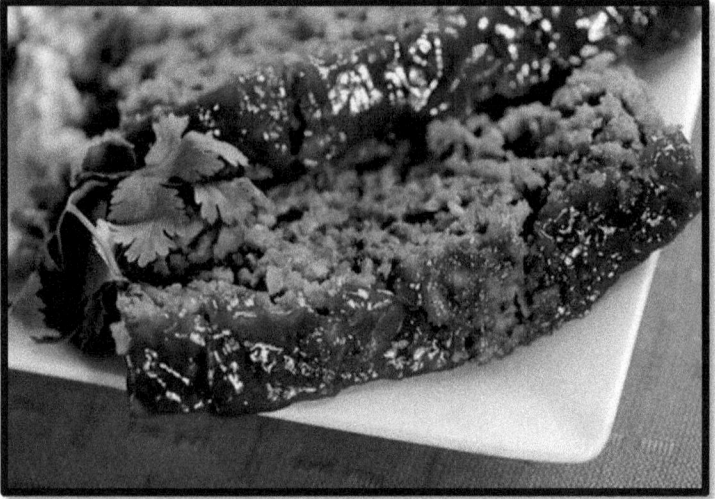

Bet you wouldn't believe that this is meatless! Even though it has less fat and calories than the traditional meatloaf, the Ve-atloaf is savory and delicious with added nutritional bonuses.

DinnerRecipes

Savory Ve-atloaf

Ingredients

1 Package of meatless crumbles (thawed)

1 Can of chopped tomatoes with chili seasoning

¼ Cup of Italian Breadcrumbs

¼ Cup ground flaxseed

½ Cup Oatmeal

2 Tbs Grapeseed oil (or olive oil)

Directions

Pre-heat oven to 375° F. Combine crumbles, oil and tomatoes in a large bowl. Mix well. Add breadcrumbs, flaxseed & oatmeal and mix until well coated. Lightly spray loaf pan or lasagna dish with cooking spray. Add mixture to pan, cover lightly with aluminum foil and bake for 30-35 minutes.

Black Bean & Potato Samosas

Ingredients

Black Beans

3-4 Potatoes (peeled, chopped & boiled)

Phyllo dough sheets

¼ Cup cooked Peas

1 Cup Red bell pepper (diced)

½ Tsp Ginger (crushed or powder)

¼ Cup Cilantro (minced)

1 Tsp Curry powder

Salt to taste

Directions

In a non-stick frying pan, heat the olive oil and add the ginger, curry powder and red peppers. Blend together. Next add the cooked potato cubes, and the peas and stir until the curry seasoned oil coats everything. Turn off the heat and add the cilantro and the salt to mixture. Mix gently so as not to mash the potatoes. Cool and use to stuff the samosas.

Thaw frozen phyllo dough overnight in fridge. Once you remove the phyllo dough from the package, keep it moist

by laying a damp kitchen towel over the roll while you work with it. If you let the dough dry out, it will crack and be difficult to work with. Put olive oil in a small bowl and clear an area on your counter to work with the phyllo dough. Take one sheet of phyllo and lay it flat. Put your fingertips in the oil and then pat the phyllo sheet lightly all over with your oiled fingers. Place another sheet of phyllo over the first one and repeat two more times.

Next, slice the layered phyllo sheets into four columns. Place a spoonful of the filling on the bottom edge of one column, and fold the phyllo dough in triangles like a flag. If the filling oozes out, just tuck it in with your fingers and keep rolling. When finished, use your fingers to brush some extra oil on the outer layer. Repeat until you run out of filling. Place the samosas on a cookie sheet and bake in a 375° oven for twenty minutes. Serve with chutney to add a spicy sweet burst of flavor if desired.

Vegetable Stir Fry

Ingredients

1-1   cups each sliced red bell peppers and onion wedges

1 Cup peas

2 Tsp each minced garlic and ginger

2 Cups Broccoli

1 Cup bean sprouts

3 Tbs Sesame oil

2 Tbs Tamari Soy sauce

Directions

In skillet over medium-high heat, cook peppers, onion, peas and broccoli in oil for 2 minutes, stir often. Add garlic and ginger, cook 1 minute, stirring often. Stir in sprouts & soy sauce, cook until heated through.

Veggie Stuffed Baked Potato w/Steamed Veggies

Ingredients

1 Large Potato

¼ Cup Broccoli

¼ Cup Cauliflower

¼ Cup Snap Peas

¼ Cup Red Pepper

¼ Cup Green Pepper

Directions

Bake potato until tender. Steam broccoli, cauliflower, snap peas, and peppers. Season vegetables to taste. Split potato and stuff with veggies. Serve with remaining veggies on side.

Spicy Red Beans and Ginger Rice

Ingredients

1 Cup Red kidney beans

1 Cup Basmati Rice

2 Tbs Ginger (grated)

1 Tsp Cayenne pepper

Directions

Put rice in pot with water 1 inch above rice. Add Ginger to rice and let rice boil over medium heat. Turn heat to low and cover rice. After 2 minutes take rice from heat and allow it to absorb rest of water. Heat kidney beans in microwave with cayenne pepper. Serve rice with beans on top.

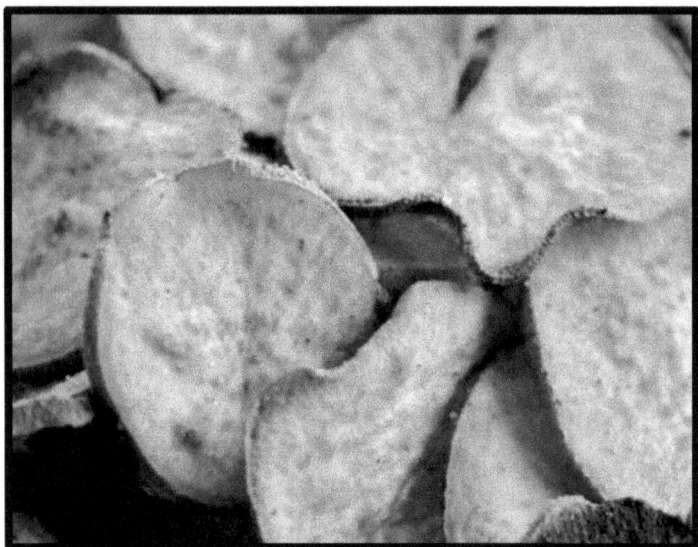

Sweet potato chips are a great snack that's packed with Vitamin A & Potassium

Snack Recipes

Protein Peanut Butter Cups

Ingredients

2 Tbs Vegetable protein powder

½ Cup Dark chocolate chips

¼ Cup Smooth peanut butter

Mini paper muffin cups

Directions

In a double boiler or a bowl over a pot of boiling water, melt chocolate chips. Add protein powder to peanut butter. Once chocolate is melted, spoon 1 tablespoon into cups. Add teaspoon of peanut butter mixture to cup. Cover peanut butter with chocolate until cups are filled. Refrigerate until solid. Enjoy.

Beautifying Trail Mix

Ingredients

¼ *Cup Raw cashews*

¼ *Cup Raw almonds*

¼ *Cup Dark chocolate chips*

¼ *Cup Raisins*

1 Quart zip lock bag

Directions

Add all ingredients to zip lock bag. Shake and enjoy.

Kale Chips

Ingredients

1 Bunch of Kale

1 Tbs olive oil

Sea salt to taste

2 Tbs nutritional yeast

Directions

Preheat oven to 300 degrees. Wash & dry kale. Separate leaves from stalks. Place in bowl and toss with olive oil, sea salt & nutritional yeast. Bake for 20 minutes or until crisp.

Sweet Potato Chips

Ingredients

1 large sweet potato (sliced)

Cinnamon

Non-stick spray

4 Tbs cinnamon

Parchment paper

Directions

Cut a piece of parchment paper to fit the glass plate inside your microwave. Slice sweet potato with a mandoline and lay slices in a single layer on the parchment paper. Spray lightly with nonstick spray and sprinkle **very** lightly with cinnamon. Microwave on 50% power for 8-10 minutes or until sweet potatoes start to very lightly brown, keeping an eye on them after about 5 minutes. Let cool completely before eating and store in an airtight container.

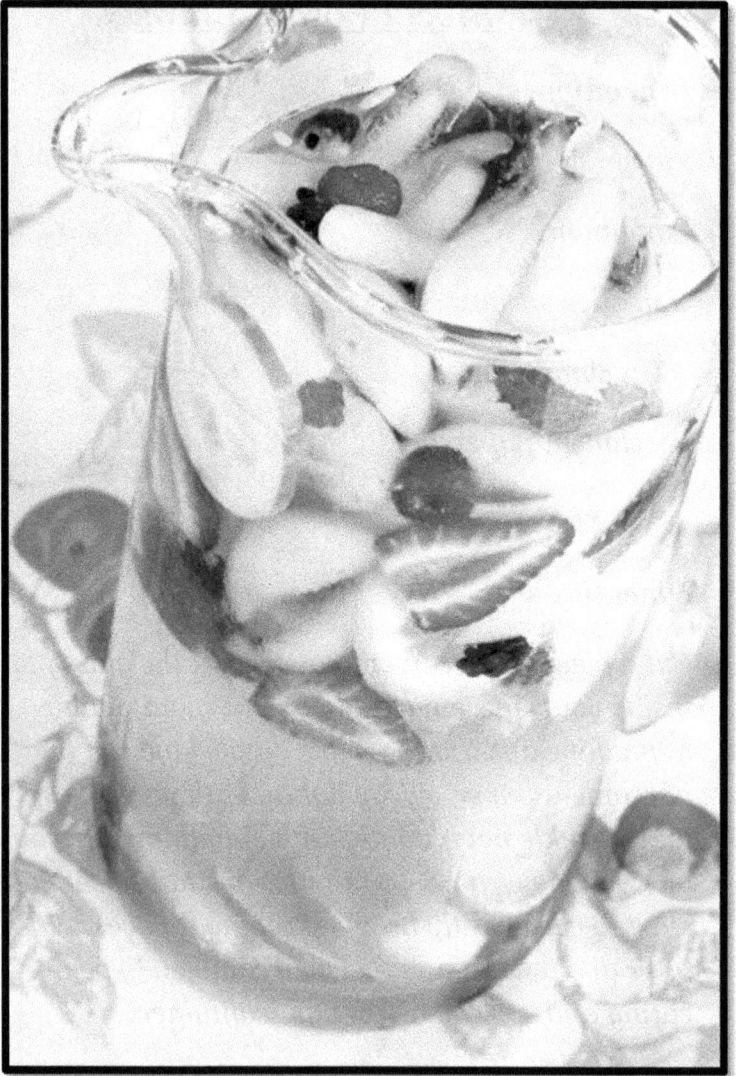

Fruit infused waters are a great way to quench your thirst while providing you with much need vitamins & minerals. It is also a great replacement for sodas & juices

Beverages

Pomegranate Cranberry Citrus Sparkler

Ingredients

1 Cup pomegranate juice

1 Cup Cranberry juice

1 Cup Orange juice

½ Cup of carbonated water

Directions

Add pomegranate, cranberry and orange juice to carbonated water. Stir & enjoy.

Vitamin Fruit Infused Water

Ingredients

1 quart filtered water

1-2 cups fruit/vegetables

2-3 tablespoons fresh herbs (mint, lavender and rosemary are great choices)

Ice

Directions

Slice fruit and add to a large pitcher. Lightly smash them with a wooden spoon to help release their juices. Gently smash the herb leaves and add to the pitcher. Add ice, then fill pitcher with water. Allow to infuse for at least 3-4 hours, though overnight is best. Enjoy!

Cinnamon Chocolate Chai

Ingredients

1 bag black tea

1 Cup boiling water

2 Tsp honey

2 Tsp cup unsweetened cocoa powder

2 Tbs Almond milk

2/3 Tsp vanilla

1/3 Tsp ground cinnamon

1/3 Tsp grated nutmeg

Directions

In a large mug, pour boiling water over tea bag. Steep for 10 minutes. Discard bag. Stir in remaining ingredients. Add peppermint stick if desired.

Important Nutrients & Their Roles

There are many foods that give us the nutrients that we need in order to have the health that we desire. These nutrients play an important role in beautification from the inside out. These nutrients also have healing properties and can cure what ails us.

The aforementioned recipes have the nutrients we need to look and feel like that fabulous naturalista that we want to be. Let's face it, we are fierce and we want every part of us to show it. It's not just about the hair, and even with it being about hair you can't have the fabulous outer without having the fabulous inner.

The following pages will give you the low down on our 'Power Nutrients', their roles and some foods that are loaded with them!

Please note that while many foods contain the nutrients that we need for a beautiful body, gorgeous skin and healthy hair, supplements may be needed in order to achieve maximum benefits.

Vitamin A

Vitamin A in all forms is very helpful when it comes to healthy skin as well as developing a great resistance to infections. You can get Vitamin A known as retinol in animal foods and beta-carotene or carotene, another form of Vitamin A from plant foods.

Carotene-rich foods are more popular than those high in retinol due to high intakes of carotene are a lot safer than large intakes of retinol. Retinol in high doses can lead to toxic symptoms, peeling skin, headaches and digestive problems, so a plant-based diet is a healthier way to go in order to get your Vitamin A, especially in large quantities as multi-vitamins or supplements almost always contain retinol and not carotene. The following foods are great sources of Vitamin A

Tomatoes	*Carrots*
Apricots	*Kale*
Nectarines	*Spinach*
Sweet Potatoes	*Broccoli*
Peaches	*Greens*

B Vitamins

B vitamins are important in many ways, one being metabolizing protein and another is promoting healthy blood and cells. Familiar names of the B vitamins include, Thiamine, Riboflavin, Niacin, Folate or Folic Acid, B6 and B12.

B vitamins are found in whole unprocessed foods.
Good sources for B vitamins are:

Whole Grains	Potatoes
Beans	Turkey
Tuna	Bananas
Lentils	Nutritional Yeast

Vitamin B12 is one to take note of as it is one of the B vitamins that is not available from plant products. For those who are on a Vegan dietary plan, supplements may be taken to ward off deficiency.

Vitamin C

There's no question to the fact that Vitamin C boasts a lot of benefits. It helps in the absorption of iron, metabolism of Folate and proteins as well as the formation of collagen. Vitamin C is also known to reduce the formation of many cancer-causing agents. You can consume your Vitamin C from these and other sources:

Blackberries	Citrus Fruits
Spinach	Honey Dew Melon
Tomatoes	Strawberries
Sweet Potatoes	Cabbage
Sour Cherries	Bananas

Vitamin D

Vitamin D is very important especially when it comes to the development of our bones. Without Vitamin D, Calcium would be unable to effectively do its job. The body would be unable to metabolize Calcium without its partner Vitamin D. Our primary source of Vitamin D comes from the sun. As the list of Vitamin D fortified foods are very limited, Vitamin D in supplement form may be the way to go to get your adequate supply.

Vitamin E

Vitamin E was widely known as being essential for metabolizing polyunsaturated fat, but has since then been acknowledged for its value in treating benign lumps within the breast. The best source of finding large doses of this useful vitamin is in supplement form.

Calcium

Calcium has always taken the front seat when it comes to nutrition. Being linked to heart health, strong bones and cancer prevention, it's a surprise. The following foods are a few of the many that contain great sources for Calcium. Remember to have an adequate intake of Vitamin D as stated earlier.

Baked Beans   Greens
Broccoli   Okra
Milk   Tofu
Soybeans   Yogurt

Iron

Iron is needed for the building of healthy red blood cells. However low iron levels tend to be a normal problem for menstruating women as well as young children. The body stores some iron, however we must build our supply daily and those in high-risk groups may need a daily supplement. Beans, bran, seeds and iron-fortified cereals are some of the foods that can provide us with the iron we need to keep our red blood cells healthy and happy.

Magnesium

Being essential to our nervous system Magnesium plays a key role in our health. This mineral helps in the prevention of heart disease and is found in bone , in which, teamed with Calcium and Vitamin D make Magnesium a weapon against osteoporosis. Eating foods from the following list can help you maximize your Magnesium intake.

Soybeans   Cauliflower
Oatmeal   Celery

Beans

Grapefruit

Salmon

Potatoes

Blackberries

Turkey

Tomatoes

Spinach

Potassium

Potassium is a major mineral that helps us keep our blood pressure in check, with the help of sodium. This mineral also helps other nutrients keep our nerves and muscles working as well as store the carbohydrates that we need. Great sources of Potassium you can find in the following foods:

Apples

Pomegranate

Dates

Tomatoes

Cauliflower

Potatoes

Cannellini Beans

Prunes

Spinach

Bananas

Zinc

Zinc is very as it helps in building our bones as well as making protein. It also affects our senses of smell and taste. Zinc is known as the healing mineral because it assists in healing wounds. You can get your share of Zinc from oatmeal, bran, lentils, spinach and many other foods.

Epilogue

When it comes to embracing our natural beauty, we must take charge so we can have what we want. When we incorporate the 'Do it yourself' method in our lives we take control and the accomplishments are greater and the failures are easy to learn from. It's empowering and believe it or not very humbling.

Keep in mind that being beautiful is not just about our outer appearance. However we know that we are visual people and that if we look good, we feel good, we do good, so when it comes to beauty and being naturally beautiful and confident, let's start from the inside so it can radiate on the outside. We do that by taking responsibility for our lives and that includes what we put into and what we do to our bodies. It also includes taking charge and limiting excuses from our speech.

Make sure you visit us at Grateful2BNatural.com for more recipes and tips. Don't forget to check out our Naturalista Nuggets page: (Grateful2BNatural.com/naturalistanuggets) as well as take part in our DIY Dares: (Grateful2BNatural.com/DIYdares)

Always remember to embrace your beauty and be Grateful 2 B Natural!

EPILOGUE

Acknowledgements

Bismillah- Of course first and foremost, all thanks and praise to the Most High! Without the Creator none of this or anything would be possible. And we know this ☺

There are so many who have inspired me through my natural journey as well as through my life transformation journey, which is one of the reasons this book was written. I was taught the philosophy to trust yourself and that no one would care for you like you can- so we must step up to the plate and take charge of ourselves and stop putting the things we love and care for in the power of others.

To my curlfriends who've inspired me with their stories and kept me in learning mode through their questions, this book could not have been written without your help. Continue to be knowledge seekers and take charge.

To my family, thank you for being patient with me through the research, hours spent cooped up in my space, movie night postponements, assisting with promo videos and all. You are wonderful and because of your love and belief in me and my project, I couldn't ask for more. Love you.

To my wonderful husband who has been my rock, thank you for pushing me and letting me know when to slow down to speed up. Thank you for the great ideas and being there as my editor, motivator, inspiration and so much more. Te amo mi amor de mi vida!

To the countless others who have taken a spot in my life and taught me much throughout my natural journey: *Chris-Tia Donaldson, *Anu Prestonia, * Khamit Kinks, *Taliah Waajid, *Isis 'Naturally Isis' Brantley, *Calvis 'The Criscokid' Williamson, *Curly Nikki, *Rochelle 'Black Onyx' Graham, *Jessica Mack, *Natasha Ford, *Donna Chase, *Chase Ford Productions, *Dr. Nina 'Beautiful Brown Babydol' Ellis-Hervey, *Denitrika 'Pretty Dimples' Craig, Malaika Tamu Cooper, Kanika Jamila and the many others who've paved the way and have shown that it's fierce and fabulous to embrace your beauty and be grateful 2 b natural.

Nyla

* Information on these naturalistas can be found at Grateful2BNatural.com/g2bnlikes

ACKNOWLEDGEMENTS

Bonus Material

Being conscious and proactive about our health is one of the first things we must do when it comes to embracing our natural beauty. Getting rid of (or at least cutting down on) a lot of the artificial 'phonyness' that we put on and in our bodies is a great start to becoming and staying naturally beautiful. Of course it doesn't begin or end with this book.

You can get training and coaching on subjects such as these:

-Water- When It Is bad for Your Skin, Hair and Body
-The ABCs of Natural Beauty
-Sneaking the Good of What You Hate into What You Love
-Burning Fat Without Cardio
-Growing and Maintaining Beautiful Natural Hair by Keeping it Simple

For this and much more, visit Grateful2BNatural.com

About the Author

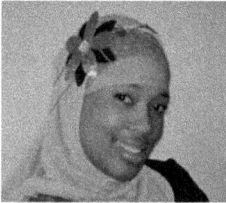

Nyla Al-Mujaahid *is founder of Grateful 2 B Natural and creator of the Natural Beauty Academy. She continues to train women and young girls around the world on embracing their natural beauty and increasing their quality of life by taking charge and loving themselves inside and out.*

An influential speaker and host of the internet radio show, Embracing Your Beauty, Nyla's books, products, articles and appearances inspire many year after year.

A wife and mother of three, Nyla enjoys her busy life with her family, friends and those she call her Fierce Naturalista Curlfriends, women whom she meet during her travels and through programs, who also share the journey of embracing natural beauty. Meet Nyla and get free training at Grateful2BNatural.com

www.ingramcontent.com/pod-product-compliance
Lightning Source LLC
Chambersburg PA
CBHW052045270326
41931CB00012B/2644